Multiple Choice Questions for Ophthalmologists

Multiple Choice Questions for Ophthalmologists

Compiled by

S. P. B. PERCIVAL M.A., M.B., B.Chir., D.O., F.R.C.S.

Consultant Ophthalmic Surgeon to the Scarborough Group of Hospitals;
Late Assistant Clinical Tutor, University of Birmingham

Foreword by K. Rubinstein M.D., F.R.C.S.E., D.O.M.S.

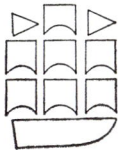

Churchill Livingstone Edinburgh and London 1972

ISBN 0 443 00905 8

Printed in Great Britain

Foreword

Anyone who has tried to put together multiple choice questions will know how difficult it is to be precise, accurate and unambiguous. Mr Percival has tackled his task with enthusiasm and has a clearly conceived sense of purpose. His inspiration came from his own experience as a candidate for higher degrees in ophthalmology as well as from his experience as one of the organisers of postgraduate teaching at the Birmingham and Midland Eye Hospital.

Multiple choice questions are probably the fairest way of testing knowledge and they can be used in a variety of ways to explore an individual's grasp of his speciality. They should not, however, be considered as a means to an end but as a tool with which the individual can assess his own knowledge and the gaps in it.

Many questions in this little book may be considered difficult to answer, but what better incentive to go back to books and further clinical enquiry than a shock of revealed uncertainty in areas which one considers home territory. I hope that this work will not only help to ease the passage through the examination net for the juniors but will find place to stimulate their senior colleagues as well.

K. RUBINSTEIN

Acknowledgements

I would like to express my gratitude to Mr K. Rubinstein, who first suggested the value of a book of this nature, for his constant encouragement and thoughtful criticisms during the preparation of the questions and also for his care in contributing the foreword. I am indebted to Mr M. J. Roper-Hall for his kind and tireless criticism during the preparation of the book, and to Mr S. J. Crews, Mr Vernon H. Smith, Mr L. P. Jameson Evans, Mr W. Martin Walker, Dr D. R. Barry, Dr A. Paton, Dr W. Cant, Dr D. G. Jamieson, Dr E. R. Bickerstaff and Dr L. Langton, all of whom have helped in so many ways during the construction and editing of the questions.

I thank the members of the junior staff at the Birmingham and Midland Eye Hospital and at Selly Oak Hospital who during the past 18 months have helped to form a pilot study in assessing the value of the questions for examination candidates. Their helpful and continued criticism was invaluable in the rephrasing of many questions, and it is hoped that they in turn benefited from the seminars which the papers involved.

Finally I have great pleasure in recording thanks to Mary, my wife, for her work in typing the manuscript and help with proof-correcting, and to Miss Paulette Oulsnan, who assisted with the typing.

S.P.B.P.

Contents

Introduction

Multiple choice questions are now a familiar feature of medical examinations in Great Britain and their use is still increasing. The oldest method of multiple choice question setting is that with only one correct answer out of a choice of five and this is still the most common method in North America. However, the method employed in this booklet is, in the main, similar to the type used in the M.R.C.P. examinations, that is, there may be one to five correct answers out of five in each question. This has several advantages:

(a) The choice is made more difficult for the candidate because he has to discriminate between right and wrong at each line rather than at each question taken as a whole.

(b) By this means it is possible to introduce misleading falsehoods against which the good candidate will discriminate, whereas another candidate, who is able to make an equally good showing on the 'one out of five' type but is not able to draw on facts from his memory quite as fast or as clearly, will be misled. This means that as a time limit is set for each paper, the candidate may find himself in an environment approximating more to examination conditions. The use of double negatives likewise calls for greater precision and clarity of thought.

(c) It is possible to cover a wider field of ophthalmology in a shorter space because each of the five lines may concern different facts relating to the same subject, whereas in the 'one out of five' type each line must relate to the same fact.

A criticism of this 'British' type of question is that absolute truth or absolute falsehood are uncommon, and that because much is written about rarities it is easy to find references which will over-inform on a point that is rare and atypical. It may therefore be that the choice of some answers is a matter of opinion; but it must also be said that in the 'one out of five' type of question a matter of opinion may also lead to ambiguity, for example, in one man's experience there may be two answers which appear equally correct. Clearly there are inherent defects in either method, but the questions in this booklet have been reviewed by several consulting ophthalmic surgeons, including two who are past or present examiners for the Final Fellowship examinations, and it is hoped that the answers which are not absolute in their truth or falsehood, will at least represent a majority opinion.

The questions have been set with higher postgraduate teaching in mind and in many cases obvious answers have been omitted. References are taken freely from the standard textbooks in ophthalmic surgery, ophthalmic medicine, ophthalmic pathology, physiology, optics and anatomy. The references listed are only those which are thought to provide useful information not easily obtained from standard textbooks. Such references include recent papers concerning new advances in thought, approach or technique, as well as certain classical or more authoritative papers of the past.

One point about the construction of multiple choice questions is that words such as rare, occasional, sometimes, several, frequent, usual and common have a limited use as their meaning is relative to the incidence of the disease concerned. Thus referring to a complication as *occasionally* found in X disease might be construed as correct if it occurred in 1 per cent of cases of a common disease or in 40 per cent of cases of a rare disease, yet it would be construed as incorrect if it occurred in 40 per cent of cases of the common disease and was seen several times a month. Similarly to say that a condition is *frequently* bilateral may be confusing to a candidate whose last few cases were all unilateral. Yet it is necessary to make these qualifications, since to leave a statement 'condition Y is bilateral' unqualified would certainly lead to confusion if this is not always correct.

It is therefore felt that in testing knowledge of features to be expected in a given situation the words 'typical' or 'characteristic' should be used. When testing knowledge of occasional associations the word 'may' should be used. 'May' has the advantage of covering a wide range of incidence but it is important to exclude coincidental associations. Firstly the association must be well recognised, and secondly construction of the question must make the relationship obvious: for example, 'feature A may be seen in (may be found in, may occur with) X disease' can include coincidence but 'feature A may be related to (may be associated with, may be a factor in, may be a consequence of) X disease' does not.

Examples of the different forms of question setting used in this book are as follows:

Which of the following developments begin to take place before the fifth intrauterine month? (p. 6). Each answer is clear cut, and each presents a fact unrelated to the others, but all concern a single aspect within the same subject of embryology. A variation is the completion of a sentence, when correct answers are those that are true statements. In the example *Tonography* (p. 9), each line completes a question concerning tonography but is unrelated to the next. These questions test ability to recall facts and the understanding of clinical concepts. Some questions demand interpretation and management of given situations, these being particularly useful in preparing for viva voce examinations. Only a few questions involve the interpretation of laboratory data.

Which of the following are true/false? Here there is a series of answers all irrelevant to each other yet commanding thought on a single subject, e.g. *Pharmacology* (p. 8). This setting probably presents the fairest choice to the candidate, and at the same time is able to cover quickly a wide range of topics. Double negatives are used in a few to heighten the discriminative capacity of the student, and in others the answer may appear superficially right but contains a fault which may be missed by the unwary. It should be emphasised that traps are never intentionally a feature of examination questions whether oral or written, and for this reason appear only occasionally in this book.

Which one of the following pairs is the most closely related embryologically? (p. 6). Here there is only one 'best' answer and these questions represent the 'one out of five' type of multiple choice setting.

Some questions combine the two methods: *In a patient with translocation mongolism* (p. 8), the first four lines question the number of chromosomes, a fifth would necessarily introduce an element of absurdity and therefore in order to prevent wastage of space another aspect of the same subject is asked.

Fit each of the complications (a) to (e) with one of the conditions (i) to (v). These questions are probably the easiest to answer because unknowns may be paired by elimination of others. They therefore occur only occasionally but are intended to afford some relief to a certain monotony from the other questions. Some pairs which are right in isolation will be found to be incorrect because they would necessarily make pairing of other items more difficult.

The purpose of this booklet then is twofold: firstly, to promote discussion among groups of ophthalmologists studying for examinations, and secondly, for the individual candidate both in revision and in assessment of his own chances of passing. It is firmly hoped that the candidate, whether studying for the D.O. or the F.R.C.S. examinations, will not only find the following pages interesting, but will be able to discover some gaps in his knowledge and so be stimulated into further reading.

The Scoring

Each question must be read carefully before answering. There may be one to five correct answers for each question. Each question scores a basic five points, with one point added for each correct answer and one point subtracted for each incorrect answer. No point is subtracted for an omission, and the person who, when in doubt, answers all questions as correct does as badly as the person who when in doubt makes no answer to a question. There are 13 or 14 questions to each paper and the number of correct answers to each question averages 2·5. The total score for each paper is 100.

Candidates expecting to pass the final F.R.C.S. examinations should accumulate a score of over 1010 on the 12 papers. The D.O. candidate should attempt to accumulate a score of over 920. The time taken for completion of each paper should be less than 15 minutes, with the exception of Paper nine, which may take 20 minutes.

Paper One
Basic Sciences

1 Which of the following developments begin to take place before the fifth intrauterine month

    (*a*) pigmentation of the choroid

    (*b*) formation of iris dilator muscle

    (*c*) differentiation of the foveal pit

    (*d*) pigmentation of the retinal pigment epithelium

    (*e*) formation of the lens capsule?

2 Which one of the following pairs is the most closely related embryologically

    (*a*) rods and cilia of the primitive neuroblastic basement membrane

    (*b*) ciliary epithelium and visual cells

    (*c*) ciliary epithelium and posterior layer of iris epithelium

    (*d*) dilator pupillae muscle and iris pigment epithelium

    (*e*) zonule and secondary vitreous?

3 The approximate protein composition of

    (*a*) cornea is 20 per cent

    (*b*) lens is 20 per cent

    (*c*) lacrimal fluid is 250 mg/100 ml

    (*d*) aqueous is 0·2 mg/100 ml

    (*e*) vitreous is 300 mg/100 ml.

4 The existence of a genetic basis for chronic simple glaucoma has been postulated through

    (*a*) studies of response to local steroid therapy

    (*b*) blood group incidence

    (*c*) sex linkage

    (*d*) its association with other diseases such as diabetes

    (*e*) studies of tonography in relatives.

5 The effects of dark on the eye include

    (*a*) regeneration of lumirhodopsin from metarhodopsin or from retinene+opsin

    (*b*) tendency towards myopia

    (*c*) shift of maximum wavelength sensitivity from 5000 to 5600 Å

    (*d*) abolition of impulses through the lateral geniculate body

    (*e*) elongation and a slight outward movement of rods towards the pigment epithelium.

6 Which of the following are correct

(*a*) no Muller's fibres are present at the disc

(*b*) Amacrine cells take part in the direct light reflex

(*c*) the tarsal conjunctiva of the upper lid is 3 to 4 cells thick

(*d*) microvilli can be demonstrated on the surface of the cornea

(*e*) capillaries of the retinal vessels penetrate as far as the outer nuclear layer?

7 Pharmacology: which of the following statements are true

(*a*) atropine is a competitive antagonist for the muscarinic and nicotinic actions of acetylcholine

(*b*) pilocarpine is a parasympathomimetic which acts at the ciliary ganglion and at the postganglionic nerve endings

(*c*) eserine is a competitive antagonist of true cholinesterase

(*d*) neostigmine exerts the nicotinic effects of acetylcholine

(*e*) succinylcholine is a competitive antagonist of plasma pseudocholinesterase?

8 In a patient with translocation mongolism

(*a*) there are 45 chromosomes

(*b*) there are 46 chromosomes

(*c*) there are 47 chromosomes

(*d*) there are 48 chromosomes

(*e*) siblings are not likely to be affected.

9 Which of the following may be used to determine whether suppression in a strabismic eye of a child aged 4 is facultative or obligatory

(*a*) assessment of visual acuity

(*b*) retinoscopy

(*c*) assessment of ability to fix on a light under binocular conditions

(*d*) the Major amblyoscope

(*e*) filters to produce diplopia?

10 Tonography

(*a*) gives an index of control of glaucoma

(*b*) may determine nature of surgical procedure

(*c*) is invalidated in high astigmatism

(*d*) is not influenced by ocular rigidity

(*e*) records rate of change of intraocular volume.

11 Which of the following are binocular phenomena

(*a*) abnormal retinal correspondence

(*b*) fixation disparity (monofixational phoria)

(*c*) false projection

(*d*) teichopsia of migraine

(*e*) phosphene rings?

12 Which of the following occur in the majority of dissections examined

(*a*) the recurrent branch of the lacrimal artery is absent

(*b*) the superior oblique muscle arises above and lateral to the optic foramen

(*c*) postganglionic parasympathetic fibres from the ciliary ganglion are myelinated

(*d*) sensory supply of the nasolacrimal duct is the anterior superior dental (alveolar) nerve

(*e*) the lower tarsal conjunctiva is supplied by branches from the zygomatic nerve?

13 Which of the following are false

(*a*) adenovirus is a DNA virus

(*b*) cytosine and thymidine are pyrimidines incorporated in ribonucleic acid

(*c*) iododeoxy uridine blocks the cytosine uptake in DNA synthesis

(*d*) trifluorothymidine is an antiherpetic agent

(*e*) interferon production is inhibited by steroids?

14 The precorneal film

(*a*) has properties of elasticity and compressibility

(*b*) is bacteriostatic rather than bactericidal

(*c*) contains a mucous phase separated from a lacrimal phase by a lipid phase (*d*) has an inner layer containing phospholipids which penetrate the surface layer of the corneal epithelium

(*e*) contains cholesterol esters in the outermost layer.

Paper Two
Cornea, Conjunctiva and Lid

1 Which of the following are aetiological factors in bullous keratopathy

    (*a*) vascularisation

    (*b*) endothelial dystrophy

    (*c*) stromal dystrophy

    (*d*) fluid vitreous in the anterior chamber

    (*e*) glaucoma?

2 Contact lenses may be useful in the treatment of which of the following

    (*a*) severe keratoconjunctivitis sicca

    (*b*) Fuch's endothelial dystrophy

    (*c*) burns

    (*d*) keratoconus

    (*e*) refractive anisometropia?

3 The TRIC agent

    (*a*) is a virus intermediate in size between the entero

group and the pox group of viruses

(b) is a cause of preauricular lymphadenitis

(c) may cause pseudomembranous conjunctivitis in the newborn

(d) in Great Britain, may be responsible for active trachoma

(e) is characterised by a cellular reaction composed mainly of lymphocytes with some plasma cells and monocytes.

4 Filamentary keratitis may be caused through which of the following

(a) trachoma

(b) sarcoid

(c) vitamin D deficiency

(d) Terrien's disease

(e) blepharospasm?

5 Which of the following are not a cause of pannus

(a) staphylococcal infection

(b) riboflavine deficiency

(c) Thygeson's keratitis

(d) vernal catarrh

(e) superior limbic keratoconjunctivitis?

6 The best donor material for penetrating corneal graft is obtained from donors

(a) aged between 15 and 60 years

(b) aged over 65 years

(c) with positive Wassermann reaction

(d) whose eye has been enucleated because of malignant melanoma of the choroid

(e) whose eye has been enucleated because of retino-blastoma.

7 In the preoperative management of levator resection

(a) superior rectus function must be assessed

(b) corneal sensation must be assessed

(c) frontalis function must be assessed

(d) coexisting convergent squint must be corrected first

(e) when coexisting epicanthus also requires surgical treatment, the epicanthus should be corrected first.

8 The cornea

(a) is more hydrated than the sclera

(b) is hypertonic to aqueous

(c) is dependent on endothelial metabolism for hydration stability

(d) is partly dependent on glucose from the lacrimal fluid for the metabolic needs of its epithelial cells

(e) is aided by the precorneal film for hydration stability.

9 Cryopexy

(a) is useful treatment for subconjunctival iris prolapse

(b) may cause retinal haemorrhage

(c) should not be applied over a vortex vein

(d) may cause scleral thinning

(e) is suitable for cryoextraction of cataract at a temperature of $-120°C$.

10 Which of the following may be associated with pigment deposition in the conjunctiva

(a) Addison's disease (hypofunction of the adrenal cortex)

(b) Hurler's syndrome (gargoylism)

(c) total hyphaema

(d) topical use of neutral adrenaline

(e) prolonged administration of chlorpromazine?

11 Increased visibility of corneal nerves is a sign of which of the following

(a) syphilis

(b) overwearing of corneal contact lenses

(c) leprosy

(d) keratoconus

(e) onchocerciasis?

12 Ionising radiation may cause

(a) epiphora

(b) scleromalacia perforans

(c) late chronic simple glaucoma

(d) massive necrosis of the cornea

(e) a retinopathy similar to that found in diabetes mellitus.

13 Fungal keratitis

(a) is easy to diagnose by corneal scraping

(b) is improved by steroid therapy

(c) responds to Nystatin and Amphotericin B

(d) may be associated with progressive shallowing of the anterior chamber

(e) is not associated with an immune ring in the corneal stroma.

Paper Three
Glaucoma, Lens and Iris

1 The Argyll-Robertson pupil characteristically

   (*a*) is small

   (*b*) is circular

   (*c*) exhibits segmental iris atrophy

   (*d*) constricts during accommodation

   (*e*) dilates well with mydriatics.

2 Which of the following field defects are characteristic of glaucoma

   (*a*) central scotoma

   (*b*) juxta caecal scotoma

   (*c*) arcuate scotoma

   (*d*) homonymous quadrantinopia

   (*e*) binasal quadrantinopia?

3 The Possner Schlossman syndrome (glaucomatocyclitic crisis) is typically

   (*a*) self limiting

(b) unilateral

(c) associated with field loss

(d) not painful

(e) associated with a closed filtration angle in the acute stage.

4 In a normal sighted eye the rise in intraocular tension following local steroid therapy is probably due to

(a) increased production of aqueous

(b) changes in the lens

(c) deposition of mucopolysaccharide in the trabecular meshwork

(d) changes in the vitreous

(e) raised episcleral venous pressure.

5 Glaucoma after cataract extraction may result from

(a) development of peripheral anterior synechiae

(b) pre-existing glaucoma

(c) pooling of fluid behind the anterior hyaloid membrane

(d) use of topical mydriatics

(e) retinal detachment.

6 A study of the developing lens shows that

(a) the first fibres are formed from the posterior wall of the lens vesicle (*b*) it is not wholly developed from ectoderm

(*c*) the anterior cells undergo rapid differentiation

(*d*) the posterior wall grows at the expense of the lens vesicle

(*e*) the lens vesicle has lost its connection with the surface by the 6 mm stage.

7 Retinoblastoma may present with which of the following

(*a*) double vision

(*b*) convergent strabismus

(*c*) anisocoria

(*d*) lymphadenopathy

(*e*) a watering eye?

8 Glaucoma capsulare

(*a*) is related to pigment deposition

(*b*) may be related to attacks of congestive (closed angle) glaucoma

(*c*) is associated with pigment loss at midperiphery of iris epithelium

(*d*) is caused by deposition of material containing acid mucopolysaccharide

(*e*) is a cause of Krukenberg's spindle.

9 Phospholine iodine may be a cause of

(*a*) stenosis of lacrimal punctum

(b) conjunctival pigmentation

(c) iritis

(d) diarrhoea

(e) vitreous detachment.

10 Diffuse melanoma of the iris first presents

(a) as acute iritis

(b) as unilateral glaucoma

(c) as unilateral cataract

(d) as heterochromia iridis

(e) as rubeosis iridis.

11 Which of the following may be the cause of leucocoria in a child under the age of 4

(a) Coats' disease

(b) persistent primary hyperplastic vitreous

(c) juvenile xanthogranuloma

(d) Norrie's disease

(e) metastatic endophthalmitis?

12 Under certain conditions monocular diplopia may be caused by which of the following

(a) peripheral iridectomy

(b) third nerve palsy

(c) retinal detachment

(d) dislocated lens

(e) treatment of eccentric fixation?

13 Cyclodialysis

(a) is used in treatment of diabetic iridopathy

(b) may be used for glaucoma resulting from a blunt injury

(c) complications include prolonged ocular hypotension

(d) should include a sweep at the three o'clock or nine o'clock meridians

(e) should be accompanied by iridectomy.

Paper Four
Retina, Choroid and Optic Nerve

1 Light coagulation may be used

    (a) in the treatment of retinoblastoma seeds 6 to 8 mm diameter

    (b) in the treatment of angiomatosis retinae

    (c) in the treatment of central serous retinopathy

    (d) in the treatment of malignant melanoma of choroid

    (e) in the treatment of updrawn pupil.

2 In choroidal sclerosis

    (a) the retinal vessels show arteriosclerosis

    (b) the pigment epithelium is deficient

    (c) Bruch's membrane is deficient

    (d) the choriocapillaris shows sclerosis

    (e) the collagen of Bruch's membrane proliferates.

3 Non-rhegmatogenous retinal detachment secondary to spontaneous uveal effusion

(a) is characteristically accompanied by panuveitis

(b) may be accompanied by choroidal detachment

(c) is unilateral more often than bilateral

(d) occurs in women more frequently than in men

(e) characteristically extends to the ora serrata.

4 Purtscher's retinopathy

(a) is associated with flame shaped exudates

(b) results from head injuries

(c) results from chest injuries

(d) is caused by air embolism

(e) characteristically clears within 1 to 2 weeks.

5 Subhyaloid haemorrhage

(a) typically has a fluid level

(b) lies in front of the nerve fibre layer of the retina

(c) may be a consequence of glaucoma

(d) may occur with any sudden rise in intracranial pressure

(e) in subarachnoid haemorrhage is due to seepage of blood within the optic nerve sheath on to the retinal surface.

6 Lattice degeneration of the retina

(*a*) is not inherited

(*b*) is found in the temporal retina less frequently than in the nasal retina

(*c*) should be treated unconditionally by prophylactic light coagulation or cryopexy

(*d*) is associated with liquefaction of overlying vitreous

(*e*) is associated with discrete yellow-white particles on the surface of the retinal lesion.

7 Which of the following statements concerning intraocular foreign bodies are true

(*a*) a localised epitheliopathy of recent onset in the lower cornea may be caused by a longstanding intraocular foreign body

(*b*) it is not possible for an electroacoustic locator to be used to determine the magnetic nature of a foreign body

(*c*) the inflammatory reaction of chalcosis may be reduced by chemotherapy

(*d*) when the media have been rendered opaque, fibre optics may be of use in aiding removal of a non-magnetic intraocular foreign body

(*e*) if 6/6 vision has been retained, forceps should not be introduced into the vitreous to remove a brass foreign body?

8 Which of the following may cause toxic amblyopia?

(*a*) tetracycline

(*b*) chloramphenicol

(*c*) ethambutol

(*d*) the alkaloid sanguinarine (Mexican poppy)

(*e*) diphtheria.

9 Which of the following may cause photopsia?

(*a*) vitreous detachment

(*b*) retinal detachment

(*c*) benign intracranial hypertension

(*d*) digitalis therapy

(*e*) chlorpromazine therapy?

10 Retinoschisis

(*a*) may occur associated with night blindness and cataract

(*b*) may be related to posterior vitreous detachment

(*c*) occurs more commonly in females than males

(*d*) typically shows retinal degeneration more markedly in the outer layers (visual elements) than in the inner layers (neural elements)

(*e*) may show strands containing vessels projecting from the internal limiting membrane in to the vitreous.

11 In 'central retinal vein thrombosis' of recent onset

(a) thrombosis of the vein may not be present

(b) anticoagulation improves the venous circulation of the retina

(c) chronic glaucoma is a predisposing factor

(d) central retinal artery insufficiency is not a predisposing factor

(e) cor pulmonale is a predisposing factor.

12 Angioid streaks may be seen in relation to which of the following?

(a) sickle cell disease

(b) Paget's disease (Osteitis deformans) in a patient aged 60

(c) Arteriosclerosis in a patient aged 30

(d) fibrodysplasia hyperelastica (Ehlers Danlos syndrome)

(e) senile (solar) elastosis.

13 Which of the following concerning choroidal melanomata are correct?

(a) shifting of subretinal fluid on alteration of posture is not a characteristic feature of a detachment secondary to malignant melanoma

(b) enucleation is the treatment of choice for all elevated melanomata over 8 mm diameter (*c*) malignancy may develop from a longstanding choroidal naevus

(*d*) malignant melanoma may present as low grade focal choroiditis with exacerbations and remissions

(*e*) lack of vascularity in a pigmented subretinal tumour may suggest hyperplasia of the pigment epithelium?

Paper Five
Strabismus and Orbit

1 Which one of the following is likely to be the most beneficial for intermittent exotropia of the divergence excess type

    (*a*) orthoptic treatment

    (*b*) treatment with prisms

    (*c*) surgical correction

    (*d*) correction of refractive error

    (*e*) none of these?

2 Which of the following forms of surgery may be suitable in the treatment of a 'V' pattern in esotropia

    (*a*) inferior oblique myectomies

    (*b*) superior rectus recessions

    (*c*) recession of medial recti with lowering of their insertions

    (*d*) recession of medial recti with raising of their insertions

    (*e*) tenotomy of superior oblique.

3 In orbital cellulitis

    (*a*) the condition is characteristically not painful

(*b*) ocular movements are restricted

(*c*) proptosis arises because of infection of intraorbital tissue

(*d*) complications include optic disc oedema

(*e*) the visual prognosis is poorer in cases with paranasal sinus infection than in cases with furunculosis of the skin of the nose.

4 In carotid-cavernous fistula

(*a*) tinnitus may be a presenting feature

(*b*) anosmia may be a presenting feature

(*c*) the patient may present with unilateral pulsating exophthalmos on the contralateral side

(*d*) carotid angiography characteristically shows pathognomonic features in the orbit

(*e*) diplopia is not a presenting feature.

5 Duane's retraction syndrome

(*a*) is not expressed genetically as a dominant characteristic

(*b*) may produce upshoot or downshoot of the globe on adduction

(*c*) may be associated with the Klippel-Feil syndrome

(*d*) is characteristically associated with retraction of the eye on abduction

(*e*) may be associated with heterochromia iridis.

6 Which of the following are correct

(a) torsion produced by superior oblique contraction is caused by rotation about the anteroposterior axis of the eye

(b) the ipsilateral antagonist of the right superior oblique is the right superior rectus

(c) Listing's plane is a vertical frontal plane about which lies the axis for rotation of the eyes in any direction

(d) movement of the eye to an oblique (tertiary) position always entails some degree of torsion

(e) extorsion produced by contraction of the inferior oblique is maximal at approximately $51°$ of adduction?

7 Blepharochalasis

(a) is associated with atrophy of the overlying dermis

(b) is often familial

(c) is associated with myopathy

(d) should be treated conservatively in young patients

(e) may be confused with epiblepharon.

8 Among the dysostoses

(a) Apert's syndrome is characterised by oxycephaly, polydactyly and ptosis

(b) the characteristics of craniofacial dysostosis (Crouzon's disease) include exophthalmos, optic atrophy and prognathia

(c) features of Goldenhar's syndrome include hypoplasia of mandible, low slung ears and notching of upper lids (*d*) hyperteliorism is due to overgrowth of the greater wings of the sphenoids

(*e*) Leontiasis ossea commences in childhood and may be complicated by epiphora, proptosis and ophthalmoplegia.

9 Left superior oblique palsy

(*a*) is rarely congenital

(*b*) causes the head to be tilted towards the intorted eye

(*c*) causes the right eye to be hypophoric

(*d*) is associated with upward turning of the palsied eye when the head is tilted forcibly to the right shoulder

(*e*) should be corrected by weakening the contralateral synergist as the primary surgical procedure.

10 A form of binocular vision is obtained by

(*a*) macular suppression with peripheral fusion

(*b*) eccentric fixation

(*c*) unharmonious abnormal retinal correspondence

(*d*) fixation disparity (monofixational phoria)

(*e*) convergence of an eye so that the macular image falls on the blind spot.

11 Which of the following are false

(*a*) optokinetic nystagmus may be obtained during the first month of life

(*b*) acuity of 6/9 is usual by 4 years of age

(*c*) accommodation does not commence before 2 months

(*d*) convergence does not commence before 2 months

(*e*) at 6 months the orbital axes are directed towards the nasal septum?

12 Which of the following are recognised procedures in the treatment of severe progressive endocrine exophthalmos

(*a*) surgical ablation of the pituitary gland

(*b*) systemic Prednisolone of a dose up to 120 mg daily

(*c*) extraocular muscle surgery, if there is persistent diplopia

(*d*) orbital decompression through the maxillary antrum

(*e*) retrobulbar injections of hyaluronidase?

13 Which of the following are characteristic features in blow out fracture of the orbit

(*a*) enophthalmos

(*b*) proptosis

(*c*) diplopia worst on downward gaze

(*d*) fracture of the orbital margin

(*e*) positive duction test under general anaesthesia.

14 Pleomorphic adenoma of the lacrimal gland

(*a*) does not spread directly into the cranium

(*b*) may undergo squamous metaplasia

(c) should be biopsied before decision on treatment is made

(d) histologically does not show sheets of spindle shaped cells

(e) may require exenteration.

Paper Six
Ophthalmic Surgery

1 Which of the following is the most frequently performed operation for congenital glaucoma

  (*a*) Scheie's cautery

  (*b*) goniotomy under gonioscopic control

  (*c*) cyclodialysis

  (*d*) goniopuncture

  (*e*) trabeculotomy under microscopic control?

2 When performing cataract extraction in a patient of 56 who has had retinal detachment in the fellow phakic eye, it is preferable

  (*a*) to perform intracapsular extraction

  (*b*) to perform extracapsular extraction

  (*c*) to perform peripheral iridectomy

  (*d*) to perform broad iridectomy

  (*e*) to use α-chymotrypsin.

3 A patient has bilateral cataract; prior to the first extraction it is thought that a retrobulbar haematoma has been caused

by an injection. Which of the following should be the procedure of choice

(a) give intravenous urea and proceed carefully with the operation

(b) apply firm pressure over the eye for 3 minutes, give intravenous Diamox, and proceed with the operation

(c) wait until the bleeding has stopped and then proceed with the operation

(d) return the patient to the ward

(e) operate on the other eye?

4 To which of the following is flat anterior chamber in a hard phakic eye following glaucoma surgery likely to respond

(a) Scheie's filtration operation

(b) intensive miotic treatment

(c) intensive mydriatic and cycloplegic treatment

(d) cyclodiathermy

(e) posterior sclerotomy and puncture of vitreous with reformation of the anterior chamber?

5 Fit each complication of glaucoma operations (a) to (e) with one of the conditions (i) to (v)

(a) malignant glaucoma (i) cyclodialysis

(b) post-operative iritis (ii) trephine

(c) distorted pupil (iii) iridencleisis

(*d*) late endophthalmitis   (iv) Scheie's operation

(*e*) hyphaema   (v) preoperative narrow angle

6 Which of the following may be associated with new vessel formation

(*a*) anoxia

(*b*) steroid administration

(*c*) oedema of tissue

(*d*) venous congestion

(*e*) infection?

7 Which of the following statements are correct

(*a*) Paufique's knife is spatula shaped and used in penetrating keratoplasty

(*b*) Lang's twin knives are used for capsulectomy in congenital cataract

(*c*) Herbert's sclerotomy knife is blunt ended and employed in filtration procedures

(*d*) a two piece corneal implant makes for easy clearing of retroprosthetic membranes

(*e*) the Binkhorst anterior chamber lens gives rise to fewer complications than the Strampelli lens because its feet are fenestrated?

8 The chance of vitreous loss during cataract extraction may be influenced by

(*a*) the type of sedation given

(b) the use of the Flieringa ring

(c) the extent of akinesia

(d) the use of preoperative osmotic agents

(e) the type of iridectomy performed.

9 A cataractous subluxated lens

(a) should be treated conservatively with topical miotics

(b) should be extracted with an erysophake

(c) should be extracted with a vectis or cryoprobe

(d) if untreated, may cause bullous keratopathy

(e) may result from chronic uveitis.

10 A 12° alternating divergent squint which becomes latent for near vision in a patient aged 30

(a) is related to convergence insufficiency

(b) should be treated with prisms

(c) should be operated on only for cosmetic reasons

(d) is likely to cause troublesome diplopia following surgery

(e) should be corrected with bilateral lateral rectus recessions.

11 A small glass corneal foreign body which is projecting into the anterior chamber

(a) is best treated conservatively

(*b*) is best removed by direct corneal dissection under local anaesthetic

(*c*) is best removed by direct dissection under general anaesthetic with the aid of a keratone or other flat instrument in the anterior chamber

(*d*) is best removed from the endothelial side of the cornea after opening the anterior chamber

(*e*) does not require an operating microscope for removal.

12 Which of the following may be late complications of vitreous loss during cataract extraction

(*a*) corneal oedema

(*b*) macular oedema

(*c*) disc oedema

(*d*) retinal detachment

(*e*) updrawn pupil?

13 In the treatment of epiphora

(*a*) a dacryocystorhinostomy should not be performed if there has been previous acute dacryocystitis

(*b*) an intracanalicular polythene tube is suitable for post radiation fibrosis of the lower canaliculus

(*c*) insertion of a Lester Jones pyrex tube is suitable for post radiation scarring of the lower canaliculus

(*d*) an infant less than 3 months old does not require

probing of the nasolacrimal duct unless a mucocoele is present

(e) dacryocystectomy alone does not reduce epiphora in cases of chronic dacryocystitis.

Paper Seven
Neuro-ophthalmology

1 A man of 40 presents with unilateral VI, VII, VIII, and XII nerve palsies: which one of the following is the most likely diagnosis

   (*a*) syringobulbia

   (*b*) thrombosis of posterior inferior cerebellar artery

   (*c*) disseminated sclerosis

   (*d*) sarcoidosis

   (*e*) nasopharyngeal carcinoma?

2 Which one of the following is most likely to be the cause of a painful third nerve palsy of sudden onset in a man of 40

   (*a*) rupture of an infraclinoid aneurysm

   (*b*) sphenoidal ridge meningioma

   (*c*) diabetes mellitus neuropathy

   (*d*) haemorrhage into a pituitary tumour

   (*e*) rupture of a supraclinoid aneurysm?

3 **Fit each of the conditions (a) to (b) with one of the signs (i) to (v)**

(*a*) basilar artery disease

(*b*) phenytoin intoxication

(*c*) myokymia

(*d*) clonic facial spasm

(*e*) Postencephalitic Parkinsonism.

(i) intermittent twitching of one eyelid for a few hours

(ii) oculogyric crises

(iii) chronic intermittent twitching of one eyelid with facial weakness

(iv) cerebellar ataxia and nystagmus

(v) Altitudinal hemianopia

4 **Which of the following are not recognised features of disseminated sclerosis**

(*a*) the junctional scotoma of Traquair

(*b*) diplopia in the absence of paralytic strabismus

(*c*) cataract

(*d*) paralysis of accommodation but with normal pupil reactions to light

(*e*) unilateral complete internal ophthalmoplegia?

5 **In Devic's disease (neuromyelitis optica)**

(*a*) women are affected more often than men

(*b*) there may be an ascending myelitis of the cord

(*c*) a paretic colloidal gold curve is a characteristic cerebrospinal fluid finding (*d*) the incidence of disc oedema is similar to that found in disseminated sclerosis

(*e*) visual prognosis is independent of the severity of the spinal cord lesion.

6 Optico-chiasmal arachnoiditis

(*a*) is most often seen in the 20 to 40 age group

(*b*) may be due to toxoplasmosis

(*c*) may be due to sarcoidosis

(*d*) is characterised by bizarre and fluctuating field defects

(*e*) is characterised by intermittent bitemporal hemianopia.

7 Horner's syndrome may complicate which of the following

(*a*) Friedreich's ataxia

(*b*) subacute combined degeneration of the cord

(*c*) posterior inferior cerebellar artery thrombosis

(*d*) migrainous neuralgia

(*e*) carcinoma of the nasopharynx?

8 In internuclear ophthalmoplegia

(*a*) nystagmus may be latent

(*b*) there is a disturbance of convergence

(*c*) nystagmus tends to be more marked in the adducting than in the abducting eye (*d*) characteristically diplopia is not present

(*e*) the most common aetiology in a young patient is disseminated sclerosis.

9 Bilateral papilloedema may be caused by

(*a*) optic nerve glioma invading the chiasm

(*b*) craniopharyngioma

(*c*) hyperparathyroidism

(*d*) hyperemesis gravidarum

(*e*) macroglobulinaemia

10 Fit each of the conditions (a) to (e) with one of the appearances (i) to (v) seen on plain radiography of the skull

(*a*) chronically raised intracranial pressure	(i) calcified foci (brain stones) scattered over the cerebral cortex
(*b*) a tumour of the cerebral hemisphere	(ii) flecks of calcium in the subcortex and basal ganglia of the brain
(*c*) toxoplasmosis	(iii) Erosion of the posterior clinoid processes
(*d*) Sturge Weber syndrome	(iv) Displacement of the calcified pineal to one side
(*e*) tuberous sclerosis.	(v) Parieto-occipital tramline calcification.

11 **A right parietal lobe tumour (non-dominant hemisphere) may produce**

(*a*) autotopagnosia (neglect) of the left hand

(*b*) a left homonymous superior quadrantinopia

(*c*) alexia

(*d*) astereognosis of the left hand

(*e*) asymmetry between left and right optokinetic nystagmus.

12 **A left temporal lobe tumour (dominant hemisphere) may produce**

(*a*) left ptosis with anisocoria

(*b*) loss of topographical memory

(*c*) macropsia

(*d*) visual agnosia

(*e*) disinhibition.

13 **Which of the following statements are false**

(*a*) a diagnosis of ocular myasthenia is excluded by a negative Tensilon test

(*b*) decamethonium sensitivity test is used in the diagnosis of myasthenia gravis

(*c*) orbicularis oculi is rarely involved in myasthenia gravis

(*d*) electromyography in ocular myasthenia and ocular myopathy is essentially similar

(*e*) myasthenia gravis may be associated with thyrotoxic exophthalmos?

Paper Eight
Pathology

1 Orbital meningioma

(*a*) most commonly arises from the optic nerve sheath near the optic foramen

(*b*) causes symptoms of proptosis more commonly than visual loss in the early stages

(*c*) histologically is characterised by 'box' cells and pseudo-rosettes

(*d*) on plain radiography may show calcification in soft tissue of the orbit

(*e*) is the most common cause of widening of the superior orbital fissure on plain radiography.

2 Which of the following are correct

(*a*) the Henderson Patterson bodies of molluscum contagiosum are intranuclear eosinophilic inclusion bodies

(*b*) Halbertstaedter Prowazek basophilic intracytoplasmic inclusion bodies are characteristic of trachoma

(*c*) Guarnieri inclusion bodies of variola and vaccinia are intracytoplasmic (*d*) the *Treponema pallidum* immobilisation test is a more sensitive serological test for neurosyphilis than the Fluorescein Treponemal Antibody-absorbed test

(*e*) yaws can be differentiated from syphilis by detailed serology?

3 Precancerous melanosis of the conjunctiva

(*a*) is chiefly subepithelial

(*b*) may show an increase of pigmentation during the menstrual cycle and during pregnancy

(*c*) is typically flat and spreading

(*d*) may be present in multiple sites in one eye

(*e*) may occur in children.

4 On examining a section of the eye

(*a*) phakolytic glaucoma can be differentiated from phakoanaphylaxis by looking at the lens and anterior chamber

(*b*) phakoanaphylaxis can be differentiated from sympathetic ophthalmitis by looking at the choroid

(*c*) sympathetic ophthalmitis in the sympathising eye can be distinguished from Harada's disease by looking at the choroid

(*d*) diabetes mellitus can be diagnosed by looking at the outer molecular layer of the retina

(*e*) diagnosis of Coats' disease is helped by the appearance of crystals and ghost cells in the subretinal fluid.

5 Prognosis in malignant melanoma of the choroid is

(a) good if the patient is aged over 60

(b) approximately 90 per cent five year survival in the spindle cell (A) type

(c) approximately 70 per cent five year survival in the epithelioid cell type

(d) good if there is little reticulin content in the tumour

(e) statistically worse in more highly pigmented tumours.

6 Keratoacanthoma (molluscum sebaceum)

(a) is related to a hair follicle

(b) grows slowly over a period of approximately 6 months

(c) regresses spontaneously

(d) contains a central core of keratin

(e) shows absence of prickle cells.

7 Pseudo tumour of the orbit

(a) may be associated with sinus infection

(b) is characteristically bilateral

(c) is characteristically painless

(d) is readily distinguished from malignant lymphoma by histological examination

(e) treatment includes high doses of systemic steroids.

8 Which of the following are true concerning retinal vascular pathology

(*a*) hard exudates result from partial resolution of soft (cotton wool) exudates

(*b*) hard exudates result from modified aggregations of lipid filled microglia in the outer molecular layer of the retina

(*c*) cytoid bodies result from hyaline excrescences in the outer layers of the retina

(*d*) cytoid bodies occur in the nerve fibre layer and result from occlusion of precapillary arterioles

(*e*) Cajal nodes are formed by degenerating fibre axons?

9 Retinoblastoma

(*a*) characteristically has a multicentric origin

(*b*) characteristically contains rosette formations due to the grouping of elongated cells around blood vessels

(*c*) may present with hypopyon iritis

(*d*) spreads by the blood stream to the bones and liver

(*e*) spreads to the brain by extension along the optic nerve.

10 In neurofibromatosis

(*a*) the nodules of the lid margins termed fibroma molluscum are due to proliferation of nerve terminals

(*b*) neurilemmomas present more frequently in childhood than in adult life (*c*) café au lait spots are invariably present

(*d*) astrocytoma may be a presenting feature

(*e*) complications include pulsating exophthalmos.

11 Vernal conjunctivitis (spring catarrh)

(*a*) has an equal sex incidence

(*b*) may be limited to the limbal area

(*c*) histologically shows hyperplasia of lymphoid follicles

(*d*) on conjunctival scraping shows eosinophils and showers of free granules

(*e*) exhibits groups of minute grey opacities over the lower half of the cornea.

12 Which of the following may be associated with pigment deposition in the cornea

(*a*) keratoconus

(*b*) ochronosis

(*c*) chalcosis

(*d*) pterygium

(*e*) Gaucher's disease?

13 Which of the following findings may be of diagnostic value in exophthalmos

(*a*) failure of water deprivation to alter the specific gravity of urine

(*b*) failure of Triiodothyronin to suppress thyroid uptake of radioactive iodine

(c) soft tissue foci of calcification on plain radiograph of thigh

(d) low serum calcium

(e) eosinophilia in the blood with microscopic haematuria?

Paper Nine
Optics

1 Symptoms of haloes and rainbows may be produced by which of the following

(a) acute glaucoma

(b) conjunctivitis sicca

(c) interstitial keratitis without corneal oedema

(d) internal reflection

(e) cataract?

2 Which of the following statements about bifocals are correct

(a) chromatism is a complication of solid bifocals

(b) prismatic jump is troublesome with solid bifocals

(c) prism controlled bifocals are useful in anisometropia

(d) bifocals may be contraindicated in facial asymmetry

(e) the relative prismatic effect is not a problem in asymmetrical astigmatism?

51

3 Which of the following statements are false

(a) when a slit lamp is focused on the eye, the slit image is said to be conjugate with the object

(b) a Maddox rod placed with its axis at 90° produces a horizontal line image

(c) the Galilean telescope has a positive eye piece with its 1st focal point in the plane of the 2nd focal point of the field lens

(d) a spectacle lens is placed in a focimeter with its front surface facing the telescope to measure the back vertex power

(e) to correct astigmatism the axis of a cylinder should be placed at right angles to the blurred line of an astigmatic fan?

4 Which of the following statements are correct concerning indirect ophthalmoscopy using a +16D condensing lens (focal length approximately 6 cm)

(a) if the lens is gradually withdrawn from the eye the hypermetropic disc appears to become larger

(b) if the lens is placed approximately 10 cm from the eye the disc will appear of normal size in emmetropia

(c) if the lens is placed approximately 10 cm from the eye the disc will appear larger than normal in axial myopia

(d) if the lens is placed approximately 7½ cm from the eye the disc will appear larger than normal in axial myopia

(e) the geometrical magnification is approximately ×4 in emmetropia?

5 The specular reflex is

(*a*) the glare produced when the eye is placed in the pathway of a beam of light refracted from a less dense to a more dense medium

(*b*) the combination of regularly reflected and diffusely reflected light when the observer's eye is placed in the path of the regularly reflected ray

Sturm's conoid is

(*c*) the image formed from an astigmatic lens at the circle of least diffusion

(*d*) the distance between the focal points of the horizontal and vertical rays

(*e*) the emerging beam of light through an astigmatic lens.

6 Which of the following statements are correct

(*a*) in refractive ametropia the anterior focal point is at a different plane from that in emmetropia

(*b*) in aphakia the effectivity of the correcting lens is increased by bringing the lens nearer the eye

(*c*) the relative spectacle magnification is at unity irrespective of the type of ametropia, if the correcting lens is placed at the anterior focal plane

(*d*) in axial myopia the relative spectacle magnification is minimised by the use of a contact lens

(*e*) the back vertex power is the reciprocal of the back vertex distance?

7 In the accommodated eye

(a) the 4th Purkinje Sansom image is inverted, real and minified

(b) the 3rd Purkinje Sansom image becomes smaller

(c) the 3rd Purkinje Sansom image becomes larger

(d) the 3rd Purkinje Sansom image is inverted, virtual and minified

(e) the 1st Purkinje Sansom image shows parallactic movement against that of the object.

8 Which of the following do not affect the angle of deviation through a prism

(a) the refractive index of the medium of the prism

(b) the size of the aperture

(c) the apical angle

(d) the angle of incidence

(e) the wavelength of light refracted?

9 Which of the following are correct

(a) the hypermetropic far point is the position of a virtual object whose image is focused on to the retina by the unaccommodated eye

(b) the power of a hypermetropic correcting lens should equal the reciprocal of the far point distance minus the spectacle distance

(c) a toric lens is a spherocylinder whose axis is curved

(*d*) a toric lens is another name for a meniscus lens which is flattened at the periphery

(*e*) when a prism is rotated, vertical lines become tilted?

10 Which of the following refractive changes are correct

(*a*) during stabilisation of uncontrolled diabetes mellitus a patient may become more myopic

(*b*) forward movement of his lens makes a patient become more hypermetropic

(*c*) myopia tends to decrease in the early stages of nuclear cataract

(*d*) iridocyclitis may cause myopia to increase

(*e*) presbyopia may be induced by Chloroquine?

11 Prisms are of use in which of the following

(*a*) the diagnosis of hysterical paralysis of convergence

(*b*) the treatment of supranuclear nerve palsies

(*c*) the treatment of concomitant squint

(*d*) the treatment of diplopia in the absence of binocular vision

(*e*) the treatment of exophthalmic ophthalmoplegia?

12 Towards the point of reversal in retinoscopy

(*a*) the nodal point of the observer tends to coincide with the far point of the subject

(*b*) the far point of the subject tends to come to a focus at the posterior focal plane of the unaccommodated observer's eye

(c) the movement of the retinoscopy reflex becomes faster

(d) the reflex becomes brighter

(e) the far point of the observer tends to coincide with the far point of the subject.

13 Polarised light is employed in which of the following?

(a) the assessment of binocular vision

(b) keratometry

(c) pleoptics

(d) use of the operating microscope

(e) fibre optics.

14 The refractive index of a medium may be determined by which of the following

(a) the Eikonometer

(b) the Rodenstock optometer

(c) reflection densitometry

(d) measuring the dispersion of Fraunhofer lines C, D and F

(e) the Abbé refractometer?

Paper Ten
Medical Ophthalmology

1 Carbamazepine (Tegretol) is the treatment of choice in which of the following

    (*a*) migrainous neuralgia

    (*b*) posttraumatic headache

    (*c*) postherpetic neuralgia

    (*d*) trigeminal neuralgia

    (*e*) none of these?

2 Which one of the following findings is the most useful in the diagnosis of early pleuro-cephalic oedema (papilloedema of intracranial hypertension)

    (*a*) transient amaurosis

    (*b*) enlargement of blind spot

    (*c*) blurred disc margins

    (*d*) loss of venous light reflex

    (*e*) leakage of fluorescein from disc capillaries on angiography?

E

3 **Which of the following drugs may cause transient blurred vision**

  (*a*) guanethidine (Ismelin)

  (*b*) chlorothiazide

  (*c*) benzhexol (Artane)

  (*d*) tridione

  (*e*) phenytoin

4 **A type of pigmentary retinopathy may be associated with which of the following**

  (*a*) gargoylism (Hurler's syndrome)

  (*b*) syphilis

  (*c*) steatorrhoea

  (*d*) macroglobulinaemia

  (*e*) rubella syndrome?

5 **Bilateral facial palsy and posterior uveitis of recent onset is likely to be due to which of the following**

  (*a*) motor neurone disease

  (*b*) Melkersson's syndrome

  (*c*) Moebius' syndrome

  (*d*) sarcoidosis

  (*e*) disseminated sclerosis.

6 Fit each part of the brain (a) to (e) with one of the disturbances (i) to (v).

    (*a*) temporal lobe   (i)   contralateral grasp reflex

    (*b*) hypothalamus   (ii) photopsia

    (*c*) frontal lobe   (iii) left/right disorientation

    (*d*) parietal lobe   (iv) formed visual hallucinations

    (*e*) occipital lobe.   (v) hypersomnia.

7 Which of the following are recognised features of Still's disease (juvenile rheumatoid arthritis)

    (*a*) painless intermittent hydrathrosis of the knee

    (*b*) erythema multiforme

    (*c*) erythema marginatum

    (*d*) cataract

    (*e*) focal choroiditis?

8 A patient under treatment for Graves' disease (diffuse toxic goitre) has unilateral exophthalmos and one pupil larger than the other. Which of the following is the most likely cause for the anisocoria

    (*a*) Adie's pupil

    (*b*) Horner's syndrome

    (*c*) third nerve palsy

    (*d*) thyrotoxic myopathy

    (*e*) topical medication?

9 **Insufficiency of convergence or accommodation may complicate which of the following**

(a) Parkinsonism

(b) diphtheria

(c) hysteria

(d) head trauma

(e) chronic glaucoma?

10 **In cranial arteritis**

(a) the aetiology is related to an autoimmune reaction to ageing collagen

(b) there is round cell infiltration around vasa vasorum

(c) the intimal coat is not thickened

(d) haemoglobin estimation and white cell count remain essentially normal

(e) arteritis of short ciliary arteries is a cause of blindness.

11 **Reiter's disease**

(a) is exceptional in women

(b) produces manifestations which can be confused with those of ulcerative colitis

(c) produces manifestations which can be confused with those of psoriasis

(d) is cured by oxytetracycline

(e) is complicated by plantar fasciitis.

12 Which of the following are features of Behçet's syndrome

(*a*) genital ulceration

(*b*) xerostomia

(*c*) episcleritis

(*d*) thrombophlebitis

(*e*) premature senility?

13 Which of the following are correct concerning fluorescein angiography

(*a*) Choroidal glow in areas of retinal degeneration is due to retention of stain in tissue spaces of normal choroid

(*b*) Disciform degeneration of the macula glows early because of leakage and the glow persists for up to 2 hours

(*c*) Hard exudates fluoresce because of retention of stain

(*d*) Ring exudates in diabetic retinopathy are shown to be centered on areas of neovascularisation

(*e*) Malignant melanoma is characterised by patchy fluorescence the glow of which slowly increases for some time after the venous phase?

Paper Eleven
Paediatric Ophthalmology

1 Which of the following occur more commonly in childhood than in adult life

    (*a*) glioma of the optic nerve

    (*b*) meningioma of optic nerve sheath

    (*c*) craniopharyngioma

    (*d*) medulloepithelioma of ciliary body

    (*e*) pituitary tumour?

2 Which of the following types of strabismus cause obligatory suppression

    (*a*) manifest right convergent squint

    (*b*) intermittent divergent squint (divergence excess)

    (*c*) alternating convergent squint

    (*d*) manifest left divergent squint

    (*e*) fully accommodative squint?

3 Mental retardation associated with a fair complexion and aphakia is likely to be due to which of the following

    (*a*) phenylketonuria

(b) galactosaemia

(c) homocystinuria

(d) albinism

(e) the fact that the child cannot see?

4 In Leber's congenital amaurosis (retinal aplasia)

(a) signs include head nodding and nystagmus

(b) the electroretinogram is normal

(c) ophthalmoscopy shows pigmentary changes soon after birth

(d) complications include keratoconus

(e) the genetic pattern is autosomal dominant.

5 Toxoplasmosis gondii

(a) is a lunate protozoon of approximately 7μm diameter

(b) multiplies by binary fission

(c) after infecting one baby is not likely to infect subsequent siblings

(d) has not been isolated from the human eye

(e) is diagnosed in the laboratory using the Sabin-Feldman dye test, a titre of 1 : 8 or more indicating active infection.

6 Following traumatic hyphaema

(a) late glaucoma may arise from iris recession

(*b*) secondary hyphaema is statistically most common at 12 to 48 hours

(*c*) secondary hyphaema is statistically most common at 3 to 4 days

(*d*) the patient should be treated with bed rest and topical mydriatics

(*e*) glaucoma associated with secondary hyphaema may be treated by paracentesis.

7   Which of the following are correct

(*a*) colour blindness is transmitted by a sex linked dominant trait

(*b*) all children of albinos are carriers of the trait

(*c*) all children of a patient with myotonia dystrophica will carry the trait?

A normal man has two brothers treated for retinoblastoma: assuming 80 per cent penetrance, there is a likelihood

(*d*) that 16 per cent of his children will have retinoblastoma

(*e*) that less than 3 per cent of his children will be affected.

8   A baby with bilateral complete cataracts

(*a*) is best treated by aspiration of the first cataract at about 4 months

(*b*) is best treated by repeated needlings of the first lens at about 9 months

(*c*) should ideally have one eye left untouched for some years (*d*) may contain viable virus in the lens if there has been maternal rubella

(*e*) will require post-operative spectacle correcting lenses of approximately + 10 dioptres.

9 In assessing a child who appears to be blind

(*a*) maximal visual acuity of 6/36 due to idiopathic nystagmus is incompatible with an unaided reading vision of N5

(*b*) altered visual evoked response can differentiate a lesion of visual pathways from mental retardation

(*c*) optokinetic nystagmus may be absent in mental retardation although the visual pathways are intact

(*d*) the electroretinogram tends to become flat in both tapeto retinal degenerations and in optic atrophy

(*e*) an absent blink reflex to light differentiates mental retardation from macular degeneration.

10 Which one of the following is ophthalmia neonatorum most likely to be due to

(*a*) pneumococcus

(*b*) tric virus

(*c*) staphylococcus

(*d*) gonococcus

(*e*) streptococcus?

11 Subluxated lens may be due to

(a) syphilis

(b) myotonia dystrophica

(c) Marchesani's syndrome

(d) gargoylism (dysostosis multiplex)

(e) mongolism (Down's syndrome).

12 The complaint of double vision in a child of 8 may be

(a) physiological

(b) the result of a recent operation for strabismus

(c) due to an intracranial tumour

(d) due to convergence insufficiency

(e) due to preoperative occlusion therapy.

13 Which of the following conditions may be associated with cataract

(a) Crouzon's disease (craniofacial dysostosis)

(b) hyperparathyroidism

(c) atopic dermatitis

(d) Lowe's syndrome (oculocerebro-renal)

(e) Wilson's disease (hepatolenticular degeneration)?

14 The correct underlying causes of the following inborn errors of metabolism are as follows

(a) cystinosis—absence of cystathione synthetase

(*b*) Bassen-Kornzweig syndrome (congenital abetalipo-proteinaemia)—failure of metabolism of the lipid phytanic acid

(*c*) Riley-Day syndrome (familial dysautonomia)—absence of homogentisic acid oxidase

(*d*) galactosaemia—absence of galactose 1-phosphate uridyl transferase

(*e*) Tay Sach's disease (familial amaurotic idiocy)—absence of hexose aminidase A.

Paper Twelve
Miscellany

1 Mumps may be a cause of

    (*a*) disciform keratitis

    (*b*) bilateral optic neuritis

    (*c*) acute bilateral dacryocystitis

    (*d*) external ophthalmoplegia

    (*e*) ulcerative conjunctivitis.

2 The Holmes Adie pupil

    (*a*) presents as a unilateral dilated pupil

    (*b*) does not affect accommodation

    (*c*) is explained on basis of destruction of the ciliary ganglion

    (*d*) is explained by denervation hypersensitivity

    (*e*) presents a myotonic element in the younger more than in the older age groups.

3 Aqueous formation

    (*a*) is achieved mainly by dialysis under a net filtration pressure of approximately 15 mm Hg (*b*) is achieved mainly by active transport of cations across the ciliary body epithelium

(*c*) is reduced by acetazolamide because this inhibits directly the transport of cations

(*d*) in the anterior chamber contains a higher concentration of lactate and ascorbate than that in plasma

(*e*) when severely impaired, may give rise to cataract.

4 Which of the following may be associated with prematurity

(*a*) high myopia

(*b*) microphthalmos

(*c*) retrolental fibroplasia

(*d*) high astigmatism

(*e*) toxocara retinitis?

5 Which of the following are correct

(*a*) the angle kappa (κ) is the angle between the visual axis and the optic axis

(*b*) the human visual axis is normally decentred to fall on the retina nasal to the optic axis

(*c*) the rabbit has a large positive angle alpha (α)

(*d*) a negative angle alpha is more common in myopes than hypermetropes

(*e*) a large negative angle alpha gives rise to an appearance of divergent squint.

6 Which of the following statements concerning anaesthesia are correct

(*a*) topical phenylephrine has no harmful effect during general anaesthesia.

(*b*) the anaesthetist should be informed of current treatment with phospholine iodide if the patient concerned is to have a general anaesthetic

(*c*) the diagnosis of glaucoma should not be a cause for concern in premedication of a patient undergoing general anaesthesia

(*d*) the oculocardiac reflex causes acceleration of the heart when the Vth nerve is stimulated

(*e*) succinylcholine is the muscle relaxant of choice for all ophthalmic operations under general anaesthesia?

7 The blood supply

(*a*) of the optic disc is derived from ciliary vessels

(*b*) of the fovea is predominantly from the retinal circulation

(*c*) of the upper lid runs predominantly in peripheral and marginal arcades behind the orbital septum and tarsal plate

(*d*) of the optic tract is from the deep optic branch of the middle cerebral artery

(*e*) of the intracranial part of the optic nerve is mainly from the anterior cerebral artery.

8 In hysteria

(*a*) the visual field to a 1 mm target may be larger than to a 3 mm target

(*b*) the minimum form sense tends to be reduced more than the minimum light sense

(*c*) the minimum light sense tends to be reduced more than the minimum form sense

(*d*) the visual fields of each eye tend to be symmetrical

(*e*) diagnosis of convergence paralysis may be helped by the use of base out prisms.

9 The electro-oculogram (light rise/dark trough ratio) is reduced in which of the following

(*a*) focal choroiditis

(*b*) high myopia

(*c*) vitelliform degeneration of the macula

(*d*) retinal detachment

(*e*) vitamin C deficiency?

10 Intracranial hypertension in young children may be a consequence of

(*a*) middle ear disease

(*b*) excessive vitamin A administration

(*c*) tetracycline administration

(*d*) nalidixic acid administration

(*e*) sulphonamide administration.

11 In Oguchi's disease

(a) the electroretinogram is abnormal

(b) there may be associated vitamin A deficiency

(c) the visual acuity is normal under photopic conditions

(d) there is an abnormality of visual purple

(e) the cellular differentiation of the retina is normal.

12 Fluorescein photography studies on retinal micro-aneurysms may show

(a) fluorescent glow because of leakage

(b) no fluorescence at any stage

(c) fluorescent staining of the microaneurysm wall without leakage

(d) fluorescence during the venous but not the arterial phase

(e) leakage of dye into the vitreous.

13 Which of the following statements are correct

(a) reverse cutting needles are not suitable for corneal suturing

(b) in keratomileusis removal of a convex lens from the corneal disc will make the eye more hypermetropic

(c) elastic fibres are absent in extraocular muscle

(d) approximately 60 muscle fibres are supplied by each motor neurone in extraocular muscle (*e*) the intertrabecular spaces communicate with diverticulae extending into the lumen of Schlemm's canal through breaks between the endothelial cells?

Answers

Paper One

QUESTION	ANSWER
1	(d), (e)
2	(d)
3	(a), (c)
4	(a), (e)
5	(b)
6	(a), (d)
7	(c), (d)
8	(b)
9	(a), (c), (d), (e)
10	(a), (b), (e)
11	(a), (b), (d)
12	(c), (d)
13	(b), (c)
14	(a), (d), (e) [Ehlers, 1965]

Paper Two

QUESTION	ANSWER
1	*(b)*, *(e)*
2	*(a)*, *(c)*, *(d)*, *(e)* [Gould, 1970]
3	*(b)*, *(c)*, *(d)* [Jones *et al.*, 1966]
4	*(a)*, *(b)*, *(e)*
5	*(c)*, *(e)* [Thygeson, 1961; Corwin, 1968]
6	*(a)*, *(d)*
7	*(a)*, *(b)*, *(e)*
8	*(c)*, *(e)*
9	*(a)*, *(b)* [Bietti, 1968]
10	*(a)*, *(d)*, *(e)*
11	*(c)*, *(d)*
12	*(a)*, *(b)*, *(c)*, *(d)*, *(e)* [Hayreh, 1970]
13	*(c)*, *(d)* [Symposium on Oculomycosis, 1969]

Paper Three

QUESTION	ANSWER
1	*(a)*, *(c)*, *(d)*
2	*(b)*, *(c)* *(e)*
3	*(a)*, *(b)*, *(d)* [Posner & Schlossman, 1948]
4	*(c)* [Perkins, 1965]

5	(*a*), (*b*), (*c*)
6	(*a*), (*d*)
7	(*b*), (*c*), (*e*)
8	(*a*)
9	(*a*), (*c*), (*d*), (*e*)
10	(*b*), (*d*) [Rones & Zimmerman, 1957]
11	(*a*), (*b*), (*d*), (*e*) [Hamburg, 1970]
12	(*a*), (*c*), (*d*), (*e*)
13	(*b*), (*c*)

Paper Four

QUESTION	ANSWER
1	(*b*), (*c*), (*d*), (*e*)
2	(*b*), (*e*) [Hogan, 1967]
3	(*b*) [Schepens, 1966]
4	(*a*), (*c*)
5	(*a*), (*b*), (*d*) [Morris & Henkind, 1967]
6	(*d*), (*e*) [Straatsma *et al.*, 1966]
7	(*a*), (*c*), (*d*) [Neubauer, 1969]
8	(*b*), (*c*) [Crews, 1962]
9	(*a*), (*b*), (*d*)
10	(*a*), (*b*), (*e*) [Falls & Spencer, 1966; Ewing & Ives, 1969]

11	(*a*), (*c*), (*e*) [Paton *et al.*, 1964]
12	(*a*), (*b*), (*c*), (*d*) [Percival, 1968]
13	(*c*), (*d*), (*e*) [Hogan *et al.*, 1966]

Paper Five

QUESTION	ANSWER
1	(*c*)
2	(*a*), (*c*)
3	(*b*), (*d*) [Scott, 1960]
4	(*a*), (*c*), (*d*) [Bickerstaff, 1970]
5	(*b*), (*c*) [Kirkham, 1970]
6	(*c*), (*d*)
7	(*b*), (*e*)
8	(*b*), (*c*), (*e*) [Sugar & Berman, 1968; Bowen *et al.*, 1971]
9	(*b*), (*c*)
10	(*a*), (*c*), (*d*)
11	(*d*) [Dayton *et al.*, 1964]
12	(*b*), (*d*)
13	(*a*), (*e*)
14	(*b*), (*c*), (*e*) [Forrest, 1971]

Paper Six

QUESTION	ANSWER
1	(*b*)
2	(*a*), (*d*), (*e*)
3	(*d*)
4	(*c*), (*e*) [Chandler, 1968]
5	(*a*:v), (*b*:iv), (*c*:iii), (*d*:ii), (*e*:i)
6	(*a*), (*c*), (*d*), (*e*)
7	(*c*), (*d*)
8	(*a*), (*b*), (*c*), (*d*), (*e*)
9	(*c*), (*d*), (*e*)
10	(*e*)
11	(*c*) [Roper-Hall, 1964]
12	(*a*), (*b*), (*c*), (*d*), (*e*)
13	(*c*), (*d*) [Jones, 1962]

Paper Seven

QUESTION	ANSWER
1	(*e*)
2	(*e*)
3	(*a*:v), (*b*:iv), (*c*: i), (*d*:iii), (*e*:ii) [*British Medical Journal*, 1966]

4	(*c*)
5	(*b*), (*e*) [Scott, 1967]
6	(*a*), (*c*), (*d*)
7	(*b*), (*c*), (*d*), (*e*)
8	(*a*), (*e*) [Bird & Sanders, 1970]
9	(*b*), (*d*), (*e*)
10	(*a*:iii), (*b*:iv), (*c*:ii), (*d*:v), (*e*:i) [Lombardi, 1967]
11	(*a*), (*d*), (*e*)
12	(*a*), (*c*)
13	(*a*), (*c*), (*d*)

Paper Eight

QUESTION	ANSWER
1	(*b*), (*d*)
2	(*b*), (*c*) [Dunlop *et al.*, 1968]
3	(*b*), (*c*), (*d*) [Ashton, 1957]
4	(*a*), (*b*), (*e*)
5	(*b*), (*e*) [Wilder & Paul, 1951; Ashton, 1957]
6	(*a*), (*c*), (*d*) [Lalla & Thomas, 1968]
7	(*a*), (*e*)
8	(*b*), (*d*), (*e*) [Ashton *et al.*, 1966]
9	(*a*), (*c*), (*d*), (*e*) [Ashton, 1957]

10	(d), (e)
11	(b), (d)
12	(a), (c), (d) [Gass, 1964]
13	(a), (b), (c), (e)

Paper Nine

QUESTION	ANSWER
1	(a), (b), (d), (e)
2	(c), (d)
3	(c), (e)
4	(b), (c), (e)
5	(b)
6	(a)
7	(a), (b)
8	(b)
9	(a), (c)
10	(d), (e)
11	(a), (c), (e)
12	(a), (c), (d)
13	(a), (c)
14	(d), (e)

Paper Ten

QUESTION	ANSWER
1	(*d*) [Foster, 1969]
2	(*e*) [Sanders, 1969]
3	(*a*), (*b*), (*c*) [Crews, 1962]
4	(*a*), (*b*), (*c*), (*e*)
5	(*d*) [Ekbom, 1950; Silverstein *et al.*, 1965]
6	(*a*:iv), (*b*:v), (*c*:i), (*d*:iii), (*e*:ii)
7	(*a*), (*d*)
8	(*e*) [Cartlidge *et al.*, 1969]
9	(*a*), (*b*), (*c*), (*d*), (*e*)
10	(*b*), (*e*) [Henkind *et al.*, 1970]
11	(*a*), (*b*), (*c*), (*e*)
12	(*a*), (*c*), (*d*) [Savin, 1963]
13	(*b*), (*d*), (*e*) [Pettit *et al.*, 1970]

Paper Eleven

QUESTION	ANSWER
1	(*a*), (*c*)
2	(*a*), (*d*)
3	(*c*)
4	(*a*), (*d*) [Falls, 1966]

5	(*a*), (*c*) [Hogan *et al.*, 1964]
6	(*a*), (*c*), (*e*)
7	(*b*) [Banks, 1969]
8	(*a*), (*d*) [Harcourt & Wybar, 1969]
9	(*b*), (*c*) [Harcourt, 1969a]
10	(*c*)
11	(*a*), (*c*)
12	(*a*), (*b*), (*c*), (*d*), (*e*)
13	(*c*), (*d*), (*e*) [Walshe, 1970]
14	(*d*), (*e*) [Harcourt, 1969b]

Paper Twelve

QUESTION	ANSWER
1	(*a*), (*b*), (*d*)
2	(*a*), (*d*) [Lowenfeld & Thompson, 1967]
3	(*b*), (*d*), (*e*)
4	(*a*), (*b*), (*c*)
5	(*c*), (*d*)
6	(*b*), (*c*)
7	(*a*), (*e*)
8	(*a*), (*b*), (*e*)
9	(*b*), (*c*), (*d*) [François *et al.*, 1967]

10	(*a*), (*b*), (*c*), (*d*) [Hierons, 1969]
11	(*a*), (*c*)
12	(*a*), (*b*), (*c*), (*d*), (*e*) [Rubinstein & Myska, 1970]
13	(*b*) [Ainslie, 1969; Tripathi, 1969]

References

AINSLIE, D. (1969). Refractive keratoplasty. *Transactions of the Ophthalmological Society of the United Kingdom*, **89,** 647–658.

ASHTON, N. (1957). Pathology of malignant tumours: eye and adnexa. *Cancer*, **2,** 599–616.

ASHTON, N., DOLLERY, C. T., HENKIND, P., HILL, P. W., PATERSON, J. W., RAMALHO, P. S. & SHAKIB, M. (1966). Focal retinal ischaemia. *British Journal of Ophthalmology*, **50,** 283–384.

BANKS, C. N. (1969). Inheritance of retinoblastoma. *British Journal of Ophthalmology*, **53,** 212–213.

BICKERSTAFF, E. R. (1970). Mechanisms of presentation of carotid-cavernous fistula. *British Journal of Ophthalmology*, **54,** 186–190.

BIETTI, G. B. (1968). Notes on the development of cryosurgery in ophthalmology. *Transactions of the Ophthalmological Society of the United Kingdom*, **88,** 79–97.

BIRD, A. C. & SANDERS, M. D. (1970). Defects in supranuclear control of horizontal eye movements. *Transactions of the Ophthalmological Society of the United Kingdom*, **90,** 417–432.

BOWEN, D., COLLUM, L. M. T. & REES, D. O. (1971). Clinical aspects of oculo-auriculo-vertebral dysplasia. *British Journal of Ophthalmology*, **55,** 145–154.

BRITISH MEDICAL JOURNAL (1966). Facial myokymia (leading article), ii, 189–190.

CARTLIDGE, N. E. F., CROMBIE, A. L., ANDERSON, J. & HALL, R. (1969). Critical study of 5 per cent guanethidine in ocular manifestations of Graves' disease. *British Medical Journal*, iv, 645–647.

CHANDLER, P. A. (1968). Malignucoma: galant medical and surgical treatment. *American Journal of Ophthalmology*, **66**, 495–502.

CORWIN, M. E. (1968). Superior limibc keratoconjunctivitis. *American Journal of Ophthalmology*, **66**, 338–340.

CREWS, S. J. (1962). Toxic effect on the eye and visual apparatus resulting from systemic absorption of recently introduced chemical agents. *Transactions of the Ophthalmological Society of the United Kingdom*, **82**, 387–406.

DAYTON, G. O., JONES, M., AIU, P., RAWSON, R. A., STEELE, B. & ROSE, M. (1964). Developmental study of coordinated eye movements in the human infant. *Archives of Ophthalmology*, **71**, 865–876.

DUNLOP, E. M. C., KING, A. J. & WILKINSON, A. E. (1968). Study of late ocular syphilis: general and serological findings. *Transactions of the Ophthalmological Society of the United Kingdom*, **88**, 275–291.

EHLERS, N. (1965). The precorneal film. *Acta ophthalmologica*, **43**, Suppl. 81.

EKBOM, K. A. (1950). Plicated tongue in Melkersson's syndrome and paralysis of the facial nerve. *Acta medica scandinavica*, **138**, 42–47.

EWING, C. L. & IVES, E. J. (1969). Juvenile hereditary retinoschisis. *Transactions of the Ophthalmological Society of the United Kingdom*, **89**, 29–39.

FALLS, H. F. (1966). Congenital lesions of the fundus. In *Retinal Diseases*, p. 129. Edited by S. J. Kimura & W. M. Caygill. London: Kimpton.

FALLS, H. & SPENCER, W. M. (1966). Retinoschisis. In *Retinal Diseases*, pp. 182–189. Edited by S. J. Kimura & W. M. Caygill. London: Kimpton.

FORREST, A. W. (1971). Pathologic criteria for effective management of epithelial lacrimal gland tumours. *American Journal of Ophthalmology*, **71**, 178–192.

FOSTER, J. B. (1969). Facial pain. *British Medical Journal*, iv, 667–669.

FRANCOIS, J., DeROUCK, A. & FERNANDEZ-SASSO, D. (1967). Electrooculography in vitelliform degeneration of the macula. *Archives of Ophthalmology*, **77**, 726–733.

GASS, J. D. M. (1964). The iron lines of the superficial cornea. *Archives of Ophthalmology*, **71**, 348–358.

GOULD, H. L. (1970). The dry eye and scleral contact lenses. *American Journal of Ophthalmology*, **70**, 37–41.

HAMBURG, A. (1970). Norrie's disease. *Ophthalmologica*, **160**, 375–377.

HARCOURT, B. (1969a). Special forms of examinations. (In symposium on the visually handicapped child.) *Proceedings of the Royal Society of Medicine*, **62**, 557–561.

HARCOURT, B. (1969b). Ocular manifestations of inborn errors of metabolism. *British Journal of Hospital Medicine*, **2**, 831–839.

HARCOURT, B. & WYBAR, K. (1969). Congenital cataract, surgical aspects. *Proceedings of the Royal Society of Medicine*, **62**, 689–693.

HAYREH, S. S. (1970). Post radiation retinopathy. *British Journal of Ophthalmology*, **54**, 705–714.

HENKIND, P., CHARLES, N. C. & PEARSON, J. (1970). Ischaemic optic neuropathy. *American Journal of Ophthalmology*, **69**, 78–90.

HIERONS, R. (1969). Papilloedema not needing neurosurgery. *Transactions of the Ophthalmological Society of the United Kingdom*, **89**, 147–157.

HOGAN, M. J. (1967). Bruch's membrane and disease of the macula. *Transactions of the Ophthalmological Society of the United Kingdom*, **87**, 113–161.

HOGAN, M. J., KIMURA, S. J. & O'CONNOR, G. R. (1964). Ocular toxoplasmosis. *Archives of Ophthalmology*, **71**, 592–600.

HOGAN, M. J., MAUMANEE, A. E., STRAATSMA, B. R. & SCHEPENS, C. L. (1966). Malignant melanoma. In *Retinal Diseases*, pp. 359–366. Edited by S. J. Kimura & W. M. Caygill. London: Kimpton.

JONES, L. T. (1962). The cure of epiphora due to canalicular disorders: trauma and surgical failures on the lacrimal passages. *Transactions of the American Academy of Ophthalmology and Otolaryngology*, **66**, 506–524.

JONES, B. R., AL-HUSSAINI, M. K., DUNLOP, E. M. C., EMARAH, M. H. M., FREEDMAN, A., GARLAND, J. A., HARPER, I. A., RACE, J. W., DU TOIT, M. S. & TREHARNE, J. D. (1966). Infection by TRIC agent and other members of the Bedsonia group; with a note on Reiter's disease. *Transactions of the Ophthalmological Society of the United Kingdom*, **86**, 291–348.

KIRKHAM, T. H. (1970). Inheritance of Duane's syndrome. *British Journal of Ophthalmology*, **54**, 323–329.

LALLA, M. & THOMAS, B. A. (1968). Periorbital keratoacanthoma. *British Journal of Ophthalmology*, **52**, 876–881.

LOMBARDI, G. (1967). *Radiology in Neuro-ophthalmology*, pp. 232–234. Baltimore: Williams & Wilkins.

LOWENFELD, I. E. & THOMPSON, H. S. (1967). The tonic pupil: a re-evaluation. *American Journal of Ophthalmology*, **63**, 46–87.

MORRIS, D. A. & HENKIND, P. (1967). Relationship of intracranial, optic nerve sheath and retinal haemorrhage. *American Journal of Ophthalmology*, **64**, 853–859.

NEUBAUER, H. (1969). Non magnetic intraocular foreign bodies. *Advances in Ophthalmology*, **21**, 1–41.

PATON, A., RUBINSTEIN, K. & SMITH, V. H. (1964). Arterial insufficiency in retinal venous occlusion—a short symposium. *Transactions of the Ophthalmological Society of the United Kingdom*, **84**, 559–595.

PERCIVAL, S. P. B. (1968). Angioid streaks and elastorrhexis. *British Journal of Ophthalmology*, **52**, 297–309.

PERKINS, E. S. (1965). Steroid induced glaucoma. *Proceedings of the Royal Society of Medicine*, **58**, 531–533.

PETTIT, T. H., BARTON, A., FOOS, R. Y. & CHRISTENSEN, R. E. (1970). Fluorescein angiography of choroidal melanomas. *Archives of Ophthalmology*, **83**, 27–38.

POSNER, A. & SCHLOSSMAN, A. (1948). Syndrome of unilateral recurrent attacks of glaucoma with cyclitic symptoms. *Archives of Ophthalmology*, **39**, 517–535.

RONES, B. & ZIMMERMAN, L. E. (1957). The production of heterochromia and glaucoma by diffuse melanoma of the iris. *Transactions of the American Academy of Ophthalmology*, **61**, 447–463.

ROPER-HALL, M. J. (1964). Surgery of trauma. In *Modern Ophthalmology*, vol. 4, pp. 1040–1044. Edited by A. Sorsby. London: Butterworth.

RUBINSTEIN, K. & MYSKA, A. V. (1970). Clinical significance of retinal microaneurysms. *Transactions of the Ophthalmological Society of the United Kingdom*, **90**, 701–718.

SANDERS, M. D. (1969). A classification of papilloedema based on a fluorescein angiographic study of 69 cases. *Transactions of the Ophthalmological Society of the United Kingdom*, **89**, 177–192.

SAVIN, L. H. (1963). Behçet's syndrome and its differential diagnosis. *Transactions of the Ophthalmological Society of the United Kingdom*, **83**, 17–30.

SCHEPENS, C. L. (1966). Serous detachment of the retina. In *Retinal Diseases*, pp. 324–326. Edited by S. J. Kimura & W. M. Caygill. London: Kimpton.

SCOTT, G. I. (1960). Orbital cellulitis and cavernous sinus thrombosis. *Transactions of the Ophthalmological Society of the United Kingdom*, **80**, 435–450.

SCOTT, G. I. (1967). Optic disc oedema. *Transactions of the Ophthalmological Society of the United Kingdom*, **87**, 733–753.

SILVERSTEIN, A., FEUER, M. M. & SILTZBACH, L. E. (1965). Neurologic sarcoidosis. *Archives of Neurology*, **12**, 1–11.

STRAATSMA, B. R., FALLS, H. F., ALLEN, R. A., MAUMANEE, A. E., PETTIT, T. H. & O'MALLEY, C. C. (1966). Lattice degeneration. In *Retinal Diseases*, pp. 155–181. Edited by S. J. Kimura & W. M. Caygill. London: Kimpton.

SUGAR, H. S. & BERMAN, M. (1968). Relationship between the mandibulo-facial dystostosis syndrome of Franceschetti and the oculo-auriculo-vertebral dysplasia of Goldenhar. *American Journal of Ophthalmology*, **66**, 510–514.

SYMPOSIUM ON OCULOMYCOSIS (1969). (Opened by B. R. Jones.) *Transactions of the Ophthalmological Society of the United Kingdom*, **89**, 727–897.

THYGESON, P. (1961). Further observations on superficial punctate keratitis. *Archives of Ophthalmology*, **66**, 158–162.

TRIPATHI, R. C. (1969). Ultrastructure of the trabecular wall of Schlem's canal. *Transactions of the Ophthalmological Society of the United Kingdom*, **89**, 449–465.

WALSHE, J. M. (1970). Wilson's disease: its diagnosis and management. *British Journal of Hospital Medicine*, **4**, 91–98.

WILDER, H. C. & PAUL, E. V. (1951). Malignant melanoma of choroid and ciliary body. A study of 2535 cases. *Military Surgeon*, **109**, 370–378.

Printed at the University Press, Aberdeen